# Code of Ethics
# and
# Professional Conduct

## College of Occupational Therapists

## Revised edition 2010

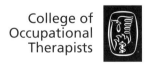

College of
Occupational
Therapists

This edition published in 2010
by the College of Occupational Therapists Ltd
106–114 Borough High Street
London SE1 1LB
www.cot.org.uk

This edition supersedes all previous editions

Author: Henny Pearmain on behalf of the College of Occupational Therapists
Category: Standards and strategy

Acknowledgements
Members of the Ethics Reference Group:
Stuart Barrow, Kate Bones, Barbara Hatton, Helen Lycett, Patricia McClure,
Jan Parry, Shirley Palfreeman, Jan Spencer.

*British Library Cataloguing in Publication Data*
A catalogue record for this book is available from the British Library.

ISBN 978-1-905944-20-0

Typeset by Servis Filmsetting Ltd, Stockport, Cheshire
Printed in Bound on demand in Great Britain by the Lavenham Press, Suffolk

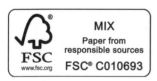

MIX
Paper from
responsible sources
FSC® C010693

# Contents

# Contents

# Preface

i. The *Code of ethics and professional conduct* (hereafter referred to as 'the Code') is produced by the College of Occupational Therapists, for and on behalf of the British Association of Occupational Therapists (BAOT), the national professional body and trade union for occupational therapists throughout the United Kingdom (UK). The College of Occupational Therapists (COT) is the subsidiary organisation, with delegated responsibility for the promotion of good practice.

ii. The College of Occupational Therapists is committed to client-centred practice and the involvement of the service user as a partner in all stages of the therapeutic process.

iii. The completion, revision and updating of the Code are the delegated responsibility of the Professional Practice Board of the College of Occupational Therapists. It is revised every five years.

iv. Under the *Health Act 1999* (Great Britain. Parliament) the title 'occupational therapist' is protected by law and can only be used by persons who are registered with the Health Professions Council (HPC). This means that they will have successfully completed an approved course leading to a diploma or degree in occupational therapy and must be meeting the current HPC standards for continued registration. All occupational therapists practising in the UK must be registered with the HPC.

v. Membership of the British Association of Occupational Therapists is voluntary. It is not a requirement for practice, but provides benefits to support practice. Members of BAOT sign up to abide by this Code, but its content should be relevant and useful to all occupational therapy personnel across the United Kingdom, whether they be members of BAOT or not. It is a public document, so also available to service users and their carers, other professions and employing organisations.

vi. The term 'occupational therapy personnel' includes occupational therapists, occupational therapists working in generic roles, occupational therapy students and support workers. It is also pertinent to occupational therapists who are managers, educators and researchers. At times this document uses the term 'practitioner'. This refers to anyone from the above groups who is working within an occupational therapy context.

vii. Where occupational therapy personnel are working in an integrated setting, or in less clearly defined occupational therapy roles, this Code will still apply in principle and should be used to ensure good and ethical practice.

viii. This Code should be used in conjunction with the current versions of the Health Professions Council's *Standards of conduct, performance and ethics; Guidance on conduct and ethics for students;* and *Standards of proficiency – occupational therapists,* along with the College of Occupational Therapists' current *Professional standards for occupational therapy practice*. The appendices to this document must be read in conjunction with local policy.

ix. Occupational therapy personnel must respect the rights of all people under the *Human Rights Act 1998* (Great Britain. Parliament 1998b). They must also comply with any current UK and devolved legislation and policies, best practice standards, and employers' policies and procedures that are relevant to their area of practice.

This version of the Code supersedes all previous editions.

*September 2010*

# Key terms

| Assessment | *A process of collecting and interpreting information about people's functions and environments, using observation, testing and measurement, in order to inform decision-making and to monitor change.*<br><br>(Consensus definition from European Network of Occupational Therapy in Higher Education (ENOTHE) 2004) |
|---|---|
| Autonomy | *The freedom to make choices based on consideration of internal and external circumstances and to act on those choices.*<br><br>(Consensus definition from ENOTHE 2004) |
| Capacity | For the purpose of the *Mental Capacity Act 2005*:<br><br>*a person lacks capacity in relation to a matter if at the material time he is unable to make a decision for himself in relation to the matter because of an impairment of, or a disturbance in the functioning of, the mind or brain.* |

| | |
|---|---|
| | *It does not matter whether the impairment or disturbance is permanent or temporary.*<br><br>(Great Britain. Parliament 2005, part 1, section 2) |
| Carer | Someone who provides (or intends to provide), paid or unpaid, a substantial amount of care on a regular basis for someone of any age who is unwell, or who, for whatever reason, cannot care for themselves independently.<br><br>(Adapted from Great Britain. Parliament 1995) |
| Competency | *Competence is the acquisition of knowledge, skills and abilities at a level of expertise sufficient to be able to perform in an appropriate work setting.*<br><br>(*www.qualityresearchinternational. com/glossary/competence.htm*<br><br>Accessed on 25.01.10.) |
| Continuing professional development (CPD) | *A range of learning activities through which health professionals maintain and develop throughout their career to ensure that they retain their capacity to practise safely, effectively and legally within their evolving scope of practice.*<br><br>(Health Professions Council 2009c, p1) |

| Cost effectiveness | The extent to which an intervention can be regarded as providing value for money. |
| --- | --- |
| | (Adapted from Phillips and Thompson 2009) |
| Delegate | To give an assignment to another person, or to assign a task to another person to carry out on one's behalf, whilst maintaining control and responsibility. |
| Duty of care | A responsibility to act in a way which ensures that injury, loss or damage will not be carelessly or intentionally inflicted upon the individual or body to whom/which the duty is owed, as a result of the performance of those actions.

A duty of care arises:

■ when there is a sufficiently close relationship between two parties, (e.g. two individuals, or an individual and an organisation). Such a relationship exists between a service user and the member of occupational therapy personnel to whom he or she has been referred, whilst the episode of care is ongoing;

■ where it is foreseeable that the actions of one party may cause harm to the other; and/or

■ where it is fair, just and reasonable in all the |

| | |
|---|---|
| | circumstances to impose such a duty.<br><br>(See Caparo Industries Plc v Dickman 1990) |
| Ethics | A code of behaviour for personal or professional practice. |
| Governance | [The systems by] *which organisations are accountable for continuously improving the quality of their services and safeguarding high standards of care.*<br><br>(*www.dh.gov.uk/en/Publichealth/ Patientsafety/Clinicalgovernance/ index.htm* Accessed on 25.01.10.) |
| Handover | To give away or entrust the total care and responsibility for an individual to another. The handover action is complete when the receiving person acknowledges and accepts control and responsibility. This is not to be confused with the role of occupational therapy personnel in a ward handover, where he or she may report information to ward staff, but still retains responsibility for the occupational therapy provided to the service user. |
| Informed consent | Informed consent is an ongoing agreement by a person to receive treatment, undergo procedures or participate in research, after risks, benefits and alternatives have been |

adequately explained to them. Informed consent is a continuing requirement. Therefore occupational therapy personnel must ensure that service users continue to understand the information that they have been provided with, and any changes to that information, thereby continuing to consent to the intervention or research in which they are participating.

In order for informed consent to be considered valid, the service user must have the capacity* to give consent and the consent must be given voluntarily and be free from undue influence.

\* see Appendix 1 for further information on capacity.

| | |
|---|---|
| Must | Where there is an overriding principle or duty. |
| Occupation | *A group of activities that has personal and sociocultural meaning, is named within a culture and supports participation in society. Occupations can be categorised as self-care, productivity and/or leisure.*<br><br>(Consensus definition from ENOTHE 2004) |

| | |
|---|---|
| Occupational alienation | *A sense that one's occupations are meaningless and unfulfilling, typically associated with feelings of powerlessness to alter the situation.*<br><br>(Hagedorn 2001, cited in ENOTHE 2004) |
| Occupational deprivation | *A state of prolonged preclusion from engagement in occupations of necessity or meaning due to factors outside the control of an individual, such as through geographic isolation, incarceration or disability.*<br><br>(Christiansen and Townsend 2004, cited in ENOTHE 2004) |
| Occupational science | *Academic discipline of the social sciences aimed at producing a body of knowledge on occupation through theory generation, and systematic, disciplined methods of inquiry.*<br><br>(Crepeau, Cohn and Schell 2003, cited in ENOTHE 2004) |
| Occupational therapy personnel | For the purpose of this document, this term includes occupational therapists, occupational therapists working in generic roles, occupational therapy students and support workers working with or for occupational therapists. It is also pertinent to occupational therapists who are managers, educators and researchers. |

| Practice placement educator | *This is the person who is qualified to supervise students while they are on a practice placement. The professional practice educator normally will have undergone a practice educators' course (preferably the COT APPLE scheme or its equivalent) and will be familiar with the assessment regulations and processes in operation at the student's university.* |
| --- | --- |
| | (COT 2009e) |
| Reasonable | An objective standard. Something (e.g. an act or decision) is reasonable if the act or decision is one that a well-informed observer would also do or make. |
| Service user | In this Code the term 'service user' refers to any individual in direct receipt of any services/interventions provided by a member of occupational therapy personnel. |
| Should | Where the principle or duty may not apply in all circumstances, by contrast with a 'must' obligation. |
| Sustainable | *Sustainable health care combines three key factors: quality patient care, fiscally responsible budgeting and minimizing environmental impact.* |
| | (Jameton and McGuire 2002) |

# Section One: Introduction

## The purpose of the Code

1.1 To be deemed as 'competent' you need a combination of knowledge, skills, and behaviours. You may learn knowledge and skills through professional training and/or experience and continuing professional development, but these elements alone are not necessarily what make you a good or safe practitioner. You must also demonstrate behaviours that promote and protect the wellbeing of service users and their carers, the wider public, and the reputation of employers and the profession. This *Code of ethics and professional conduct* describes a set of professional behaviours and values that the British Association of Occupational Therapists expects its members to abide by, and believe all occupational therapy personnel should follow.

   1.1.1 The Health Professions Council (HPC) has overall responsibility for ensuring that all relevant health professionals meet certain given standards in order to be registered to practise in the United Kingdom. Their current *Standards of conduct, performance and ethics* and current *Standards of proficiency – occupational therapists* explain these requirements. If a formal complaint is made about an occupational therapist, the Health Professions Council will take account of whether their own standards have been met, and will also take account of any guidance or codes of practice produced by professional membership bodies (HPC 2008, p15).

1.1.2    You have a responsibility to act in a professional and ethical manner at all times. The Code provides a set of behaviours and values that are relevant to you, irrespective of where you work or your level of experience. The Code, along with the College of Occupational Therapists' current professional standards and the HPC's current standards, provides you with a framework for promoting and maintaining good and safe professional behaviour and practice in occupational therapy.

1.1.3    You should be familiar with the content of the Code and should apply it in your workplace. As a practical document, it should be the first point of reference for you if you have a dilemma related to professional or ethical conduct.

1.1.4    Higher Education Institutions will use the Code early in students' education, to inform them of the required standards of ethics and conduct that occupational therapy personnel are expected to uphold during their academic and professional lives, emphasising its application from point of entry to the programme to the end of their professional career.

1.1.5    The Code may also be used by others outside the profession to determine the measure of ethical and professional conduct expected of you. The College encourages recognition of the Code by other individuals, organisations and institutions who are involved with the profession, including employers and commissioners.

1.1.6   The Code is a broad document and cannot provide detailed answers to all the specific professional or ethical dilemmas that you might face in your work. If there is uncertainty or dispute as to the interpretation or application of the Code, enquiries shall be referred in the first instance to the Head of Professional Practice at the College of Occupational Therapists, who may then pass it on to the College's Professional Practice Board.

## Defining occupational therapy, its values and beliefs

1.2   Occupational therapy has a unique approach to service users. Its beliefs and values have been drawn together and incorporated into the *College of Occupational Therapists' curriculum guidance for pre-registration education* (COT 2009d):

> *Occupational therapists view people as occupational beings. People are intrinsically active and creative, needing to engage in a balanced range of activities in their daily lives in order to maintain health and wellbeing. People shape, and are shaped by, their experiences and interactions with their environments. They create identity and meaning through what they do and have the capacity to transform themselves through premeditated and autonomous action.*

*The purpose of occupational therapy is to enable people to fulfil, or to work towards fulfilling, their potential as occupational beings. Occupational therapists promote function, quality of life and the realisation of potential in people who are experiencing occupational deprivation, imbalance or alienation. They believe that activity can be an effective medium for remediating dysfunction, facilitating adaptation and recreating identity.*

(COT 2009d, p1)

A shorter definition for occupational therapy was adopted by the College of Occupational Therapists' Council in January 2004. Listed as the current BAOT/ UK definition on the World Federation of Occupational Therapists website, it reads:

*Occupational therapy enables people to achieve health, well being and life satisfaction through participation in occupation.*

(COT 2004)

Further descriptions of occupational therapy and its values and beliefs are available from the COT/BAOT Briefing *Definitions and core skills for occupational therapy* (COT 2009b), *Occupational therapy defined as a complex intervention* (Creek 2003), *The value of occupational therapy and its contribution to adult social service users and their carers* (COT et al 2008) and *From interface to integration: a strategy for modernising occupational therapy services in local health and social care communities. A consultation.* (COT 2002).

# Section Two: Service user welfare and autonomy

## Duty of care

2.1 A duty of care arises where there is a sufficiently close relationship between two parties, as with a member of occupational therapy personnel and a service user, and where it is reasonably foreseeable that the actions of one party could, if carelessly performed, cause harm or loss to the other party. Discharging the duty of care requires you to perform your occupational duties to the standard of a reasonably skilled and careful practitioner.

### 2.1.1 Discharging the duty of care

In practice, a duty of care arises when a referral has been received by an occupational therapy service or practitioner. The duty of care would require you to assess the suitability of the potential service user for occupational therapy with reasonable care and skill, following usual and approved occupational therapy practice.

If, as a result of the initial assessment, the individual is not suitable for the receipt of occupational therapy services, then no further duty of care arises other than to inform the referrer of the decision that has been made.

2.1.2     You are required to ensure that all reasonable steps are taken to ensure the health, safety and welfare of any person involved in any activity for which you are responsible. This might be a service user, a carer, another member of staff or a member of the public (Great Britain. Parliament 1974).

### 2.1.3    Breach of duty of care

You may be in breach of your duties to take care if it can be shown that you have failed to perform your professional duties to the standard expected of a reasonably skilled occupational therapy practitioner.

### 2.1.4    Defences

If it is asserted that you have, in the performance of your duties, breached your duty of care to a service user, it is a good defence to show that a responsible body of like practitioners would have acted in the same way: the 'Bolam Principle'. The Bolam Principle will only be a good defence however if it can be shown that the body of opinion relied on has a logical basis and is respectable, responsible and reasonable in its own right: the 'Bolitho Principle'.

## Welfare

2.2   You must always recognise the human rights of service users and act in their best interests.

2.2.1   You should enable individuals to preserve their individuality, self-respect, dignity, privacy, autonomy and integrity.

2.2.2   You must not engage in, or support, any behaviour that causes any unnecessary mental or physical distress. Such behaviour includes neglect and indifference to pain.

2.2.3   You must protect and safeguard the interests of vulnerable people in your care or with whom you have contact in the course of your professional duties. Your duty of care extends to raising concerns, with your manager or an appropriate alternative person, about any service user or carer who may be at risk in any way. Local policy should be followed.

2.2.4   You must always provide adequate information to a service user in order for them to provide informed consent. This is particularly important where any intervention may cause pain or distress. Every effort should be made to ensure that the service user understands the nature, purpose and likely effect of the intervention before it is undertaken (see section 2.3 on mental capacity and informed consent, and also Appendix 2 on informed consent).

2.2.5   You must make every effort not to leave a service user in pain or distress following intervention. Professional judgement and experience should be used to assess the level of pain, distress or risk and appropriate action should be taken if necessary. Advice should be sought when required.

2.2.6 You should communicate honestly, openly and in a professional manner with service users, their families and carers, addressing concerns co-operatively should they arise and receiving feedback. Advice should be sought when required and local policy followed.

2.2.7 You must take appropriate precautions to protect service users, their carers and their families, and yourself from infection in relation to personal, equipment and environmental cleanliness. Local infection control guidance and policy should be followed.

2.2.8 Everyone has a responsibility to safeguard children, young people and vulnerable adults. Should you witness, or have reason to believe that a service user has been the victim of, dangerous, abusive, discriminatory or exploitative behaviour or practice, you must notify a line manager or other prescribed person, seeking the service user's consent where possible, and using local procedures where available.

2.2.9 If you witness, or have reason to believe, that a service user has been the victim of abuse in your workplace, you may notify your line manager or other prescribed person. The *Public Interest Disclosure Act (PIDA) 1998* (Great Britain. Parliament 1998c) places no obligation on you to make a disclosure, or 'whistle-blow'. However, such a disclosure would be a 'protected disclosure', so you would not suffer detriment as a result of making the disclosure.

2.2.10 If you are an employer or supplier of personnel, you must report to the Independent Safeguarding Authority any person who has been removed from work because of their behaviour, where that behaviour may meet any of the criteria for the individual to be barred from working with children or vulnerable adults (Great Britain. Parliament 2006, section 36).

See also standards 1, 7 and 11 of the HPC (2008) *Standards of conduct, performance and ethics.*

## Mental capacity and informed consent

2.3 You have a continuing duty to respect and uphold the autonomy of service users, encouraging and enabling choice and partnership-working in the occupational therapy process.

The law on mental capacity is set out in the *Mental Capacity Act 2005* (Great Britain. Parliament 2005) and the associated *Mental Capacity Act 2005 code of practice* (Department for Constitutional Affairs 2007). Those acting in a professional capacity for, or in relation to, a person who lacks capacity are legally required to have regard to the relevant sections of the *code of practice*. You should, therefore, be familiar with the Act and the *code of practice* (see Appendix 2). Practitioners in devolved countries should be aware of their country equivalent legislation and its implications for their practice.

You must assess service users' mental capacity to make decisions in relation to occupational therapy provision, in accordance with the provisions of the *Mental Capacity Act* 2005 (Great Britain. Parliament 2005). If the service user does have capacity, you must seek the service user's informed consent to treatment (see Appendix 2). If the service user does not have capacity, you must consider whether the proposed treatment is in the service user's best interests, having taken into account the factors and consultation requirements of the Act, before commencing treatment.

2.3.1   Where service users have mental capacity, they have a right to make informed choices and decisions about their future and the care and intervention that they receive. If possible, such choices should be respected, even when in conflict with professional opinion.

2.3.2   For consent to be valid, it must be given voluntarily by an appropriately informed person who has the capacity to consent to the intervention in question (DH 2009, chapter 1, section 1). The gaining of consent, whether verbal or written, must be recorded.

2.3.3   Service users with capacity should be given sufficient information, in an appropriate manner, to enable them to give consent to any proposed intervention(s) concerning them. They should be able to understand the nature and purpose of the proposed intervention(s), including any possible risks involved.

2.3.4　Where possible the need, or a reasonable request, to be treated, seen or visited by a practitioner with specific characteristics should be met, for example by a professional and not a student, by a male or female practitioner, or by a particular language speaker.

2.3.5　Where a service user's capacity to give informed consent is restricted or absent, you should, as far as possible, ascertain and respect their preferences and wishes, at all times seeking to act in their best interests. All decisions and actions taken must be documented (see Appendix 2).

2.3.6　Most service users have the right to refuse any intervention at any time in the occupational therapy process. This must be respected and recorded in the care record. You must not coerce or put undue pressure on a service user to accept intervention, but must inform them of any possible risk or consequence of refusing treatment. For service users without capacity, a 'best interests' decision is required.

See Appendices 1 and 2 for further guidance on mental capacity and informed consent.

See also standard 9 of the HPC (2008) *Standards of conduct, performance and ethics.*

## Confidentiality

2.4　You are obliged to safeguard confidential information relating to service users at all times. This includes when communicating with others via any medium. It is also established law that confidential personal information must be protected and a failure to do so can lead to a fine, or give the service user a cause of action for breach of confidence.

2.4.1   You must make yourself aware of your legal responsibilities under the *Data Protection Act 1998,* the *Human Rights Act 1998* and the *Mental Capacity Act 2005* (Great Britain. Parliament 1998a, 1998b, 2005) (see Appendix 3).

2.4.2   You must keep all records securely, making them available only to those who have a legitimate right or need to see them.

2.4.3   The disclosure of confidential information regarding the service user's diagnosis, treatment, prognosis or future requirements is only possible where: the service user gives consent (expressed or implied); there is legal justification (by statute or court order); or it is considered to be in the public interest in order to prevent serious harm, injury or damage to the service user or to any other person. Local procedures should be followed.

2.4.4   You must adhere to local and national policies regarding confidentiality in the storage and electronic transfer of information (including records, faxes and e-mails) at all times.

2.4.5   You must grant access to records by service users in accordance with the *Data Protection Act 1998*, the *Access to Health Records Act 1990* and the *Freedom of Information Act 2000* (Great Britain. Parliament 1998a, 1990,

2000) (or relevant/equivalent country regulations or orders). Reference should be made to current guidance (both local and national) on access to personal health and social care information.

2.4.6 You must obtain and record consent prior to using visual, oral or written material relating to service users outside of their care situation, e.g. for learning/teaching purposes. Service user confidentiality and choice must be observed in this circumstance.

2.4.7 Discussions with or concerning a service user should be held in a location and manner appropriate to the protection of the service user's right to confidentiality and privacy.

More information on confidentiality is available in Appendix 3 and from the College of Occupational Therapists' guidance *Record Keeping* (COT 2010).

See also standard 2 of the HPC (2008) *Standards of conduct, performance and ethics.*

# Section Three: Service provision

## Equality

3.1 You must care for all service users in a fair and just manner, always acting in accordance with human rights, legislation and in the service user's best interests.

    3.1.1   You must offer equal access to services without bias or prejudice on the basis of age, gender, race, nationality, colour, faith, sexual orientation, level of ability or position in society. Practice should at all times be centred on the service user (HPC 2008, standard 1).

    3.1.2   You should be aware of and sensitive to how the above factors affect service users' cultural and lifestyle choices, incorporating this into any service planning, individual assessment and/or intervention where possible.

    3.1.3   You must report in writing to your employing authority, at the earliest date in your employment, any religious and/or cultural beliefs that would influence how you carry out your duties. You should explore ways in which you can avoid placing an unreasonable burden on colleagues because of this. This does not affect your duties, as set out in sections 3.1.1

and 3.1.2, and you must always provide service users with full, unbiased information.

## Resources

3.2 Occupational therapy services should be centred on the service user and their carer(s), but local, national and environmental resources for care are not infinite. At times priorities will have to be identified and choices will have to be made, whilst complying with legal requirements, and national and/or local policy.

3.2.1 In establishing priorities and providing services, service user and carer choice should be taken into account, and implemented wherever reasonably possible. If the service user lacks the mental capacity to identify his or her preferences, occupational therapy personnel must act in the service user's best interests (see Appendix 1 for more information on mental capacity).

3.2.2 You should work as cost-effectively and efficiently as possible in order to sustain resources.

3.2.3 You have a duty to report and provide evidence on resource and service deficiencies that may endanger the health and safety of service users and carers to the relevant service manager (Great Britain. Parliament 1998c, section 43B, point (1)d). Local policy should be followed. Service managers should then take appropriate action.

3.2.4    Where the service user's or their carer's choice cannot be met by the occupational therapy service, you should explain this to the service user/carer. You may provide information as to different service providers, sources of funding etc. Provided that you have referred the service user to another agency if appropriate; complied with all the necessary procedures; and ensured that a follow up is not reasonably required, you will have no further responsibility or liability.

## The occupational therapy process

3.3    You must have and abide by clearly documented procedures and criteria for your service(s).

3.3.1    You should be aware of the standards and requirements of the professional body and the registration body, abiding by them as required by registration and/or membership.

3.3.2    You should work in partnership with the service user and their carer(s), throughout the care process, respecting their choices and wishes and acting in the service user's best interests at all times.

3.3.3    Following receipt of a referral for occupational therapy, the legal responsibility and liability for any assessment and possible intervention provided by occupational therapy lies with the occupational therapy service to which the case is allocated, even if that assessment or possible intervention has been requested by another professional (see section 2.1.1).

Code of ethics and professional conduct

3.3.4   You have the right to refuse to provide any intervention that you believe would be harmful to a service user, or that would not be clinically justified, even if requested by another professional. The guidance given by the Court of Appeal in the case of R (Burke) v. General Medical Council (Official Solicitor and others intervening) (2005), is that if a form of treatment is not clinically indicated, a practitioner is under no legal obligation to provide it although he or she should seek a second opinion. Similarly, a doctor who is responsible for a service user may instruct a therapist not to carry out certain forms of treatment if he or she believes them to be harmful to the service user (Department of Health 1977).

3.3.5   Any advice or intervention provided should be based upon the most recent evidence available, best practice, or local/national guidelines and protocols.

3.3.6   A service user can decide not to follow all or part of the practitioner's recommendations, seeking intervention, equipment or advice elsewhere. This must be recorded in the care record, together with your assessment that the service user has the capacity to make such a decision (see Appendix 2 and also point 2.3.6). Provided that you have referred the service user to another agency if appropriate, complied with all the necessary procedures, and ensured that a follow-up is not reasonably required, you will have no further responsibility or liability.

# Risk management

3.6 Risk management is an intrinsic part of governance and the provision of a quality service. Risk management is a process of identifying and adequately reducing the likelihood and impact of any kind of incident occurring that might cause harm. The principles remain the same whether the potential harm is to people, organisations or the environment. The process also enables positive risks to be taken with service users in a safe and appropriate way.

3.6.1 You must familiarise yourself with the risk management legislation that is relevant to your practice, and with your own local risk management procedures.

3.6.2 You are responsible for assessing and managing the identified risks involved in providing care to your service users.

3.6.3 You are expected to co-operate with your employers in meeting the requirements of legislation and local policy. You must also take reasonable care for your own health and safety and that of others who may be affected by what you do, or do not do (Great Britain. Parliament 1974, section 7).

3.6.4 You must ensure that you remain up to date in all your statutory training related to risk management, health and safety, and moving and handling.

More information is available from the College of Occupational Therapists current guidance on risk management.

# Record keeping

3.7 Record keeping is core to the provision of good quality and safe care. The key purpose of records is to facilitate the care and support of a service user. It is essential to provide and maintain a written record of all that has been done for/with or in relation to a service user, including the clinical reasoning behind the care planning and provision.

    3.7.1 You must accurately, legibly and contemporaneously record all information related to your involvement with the service user, in line with the standards of the Health Professions Council, the College of Occupational Therapists and local policy. Any record must be clearly dated and attributable to the person making the entry (HPC 2008, standard 10).

    3.7.2 You must ensure that you meet any legal requirements regarding confidentiality in record keeping (see section 2.4).

More information is available from the current College of Occupational Therapists' *Professional standards for occupational therapy practice* and guidance on *Record keeping* (COT 2010).

# Section Four: Personal/ professional integrity

## Personal integrity

4.1 The highest standards of personal integrity are expected of occupational therapy personnel. You must not engage in any criminal or otherwise unlawful, or unprofessional behaviour that would bring the profession into disrepute (HPC 2008, standard 3).

4.1.1 You must always conduct and present yourself in a professional manner whilst in your work role. You should act and dress appropriately to the setting, conforming to local policy and in accordance with health and safety requirements.

4.1.2 You should adhere to statutory and local policies at all times.

4.1.3 You must inform the regulatory body and/or their employers if you are convicted of a criminal offence, receive a conditional discharge for an offence, or if you accept a police caution (HPC 2008, standard 4).

4.1.4 You must inform the regulatory body if you are disciplined, suspended or placed under a practice restriction by an employer because of concerns about your conduct or competence (HPC 2008, standard 4).

4.1.5   You should co-operate with any investigation or formal enquiry into your own professional conduct, the conduct of another worker or the treatment of a service user, where appropriate.

More information on informing the regulatory body is available from *Guidance on health and character: a guide for applicants and registrants on how we consider information they declare* (HPC 2009b).

## Relationships with service users

4.2   You should foster appropriate therapeutic relationships with your service users in a transparent, ethical and impartial way, centred on the needs and choices of the service user and their family/carers.

4.2.1   It is unethical for you to enter into relationships that would impair your judgement and objectivity and/or which would give rise to the advantageous or disadvantageous treatment of a service user.

4.2.2   You must not enter into relationships that exploit service users sexually, physically, emotionally, financially, socially or in any other manner.

4.2.3   You must not exploit any professional relationship for any form of personal gain or benefit.

Section Four: Personal/professional integrity

4.2.4    You should avoid entering into a close personal relationship with a current service user. You are responsible for maintaining an appropriate professional relationship. If there is a risk that the professional boundary may be broken, this should be disclosed and discussed with your service manager. You should hand over therapy care for the service user to an appropriate professional colleague.

4.2.5    In the case of relationships, sexual or otherwise, regardless of when the professional relationship may have started or ended, or however consensual it may have been, it will always be your responsibility to prove that you have not exploited the vulnerability of the service user and/or his or her carer, should concerns be raised.

4.2.6    As far as is reasonably practical, you should not enter into a professional relationship with someone with whom you already have, or have had, a close personal relationship. This includes family members and friends. Where there is no reasonable alternative, you must make every effort to remain professional and objective whilst working with the individual you know or have known.

4.2.7    In such circumstances this should be disclosed and discussed with the service manager and a note should be made in care records. This is for your protection as much as for the service user.

More information is available concerning sexual relationships and boundaries from the COT/BAOT

Briefing *Clear sexual boundaries between healthcare professionals and patients: responsibilities of healthcare professionals* (COT 2009a).

## Professional integrity

4.3 You must act with honesty and integrity at all times. You must not get involved in any behaviour or activity that is likely to damage the public's confidence in you or your profession.

(HPC 2008, standard 13)

4.3.1 You must adhere to statutory and local policies with regard to discrimination, bullying and harassment.

4.3.2 Any reference to the quality of work, or the integrity of a professional colleague should be expressed with due care to protect the reputation of that person. Any opinion must be evidence-based and given through appropriate channels. When providing a second opinion to a service user and/or their carer, it must be confined to the case in question and not extend to the general competence of the first practitioner.

4.3.3 Should you have reasonable grounds to believe that the behaviour or professional performance of a colleague may be deficient in standards of professional competence, you should notify the line manager or other appropriate person in strictest confidence. This includes (but is not limited to) when a colleague's performance is seriously deficient, when he or she has a health problem which is impairing his or her competence to practise, or when he or she is practising in a manner which places service users or colleagues at risk.

4.3.4   In reporting any concerns to a line manager or other appropriate person, the information must be objective, relevant and limited to the matter of concern.

4.3.5   Under no circumstances should you remain silent about any malpractice, criminal conduct or unprofessional activity that you witness, whether by occupational therapy personnel or other staff.

4.3.6   You may give evidence in court concerning any alleged negligence of a colleague. Such evidence must be objective and capable of substantiation.

## Fitness to practise

4.4   You must inform your employer/appropriate authority and the Health Professions Council about any health or personal conditions that may affect your ability to perform your job competently and safely.

4.4.1   You should limit or stop working if your performance or judgement is affected by your health (HPC 2008, standard 12).

## Substance misuse

4.5   You must not undertake any professional activities whatsoever when under the influence of alcohol, drugs or other intoxicating substances.

4.5.1   You must not promote and/or use illegal substances in the workplace.

## Personal profit or gain

4.6   You should not accept tokens such as favours, gifts or hospitality from service users, their families or commercial organisations when this might be construed as seeking to obtain preferential treatment (Great Britain. Parliament 1889, 1906, 1916). In respect of private practice this principle still prevails in terms of personal gain.

4.6.1   Local policy should always be observed in the case of gifts.

4.6.2   If a service user or their family makes a bequest to a practitioner or a service, this should be declared according to local guidelines.

4.6.3   You must put the interests of the service user first and should not let this duty be influenced by any commercial or other interest that conflicts with this duty, for example in arrangements with commercial providers that may influence contracting for the provision of equipment.

## Information and representation

4.7   Information and/or advertising, in respect of professional activities or work, must be accurate. It should not be misleading, unfair or sensational (HPC 2008, standard 14).

4.7.1 You should accurately represent your qualifications, education, experience, training, competence and the services you provide. Explicit claims should not be made in respect of superiority of personal skills, equipment or facilities.

4.7.2 You should not claim another person's work or achievements as your own unless the claim can be fully justified. You should respect the intellectual property rights of others at all times.

4.7.3 You may only advertise, promote or recommend a product or service in an accurate and objective way. You may not support or make unjustifiable statements about a product or service.

4.7.4 If you are aware that possible misrepresentation of the protected title 'occupational therapist' has occurred, you must contact the Health Professions Council.

# Section Five: Professional competence and lifelong learning

## Professional competence

5.1 You must only provide services and use techniques for which you are qualified by education, training and/or experience. These must be within your professional competence, appropriate to the needs of the service user and relate to your terms of employment.

   5.1.1   You should achieve and continuously maintain high standards in your professional knowledge, skills and behaviour.

   5.1.2   You should be aware of and abide by the current legislation, guidance and standards that are relevant to your practice.

   5.1.3   If you are asked to act up or cover for an absent colleague, such duties should only be undertaken with additional planning, support, supervision and/or training. You should be able to refuse such a request, without reprisal, if you believe the work to be outside the scope of your competence or workload capacity.

5.1.4    If you are seeking to work in areas with which you are unfamiliar or in which your experience has not been recent, you should ensure that adequate self-directed learning takes place as well as other relevant training and supervision.

5.1.5    If you extend your role beyond the scope of occupational therapy practice, or if you take on a new role, you must ensure that additional skills are acquired and maintained for safe and competent practice, for example in prescribing (COT 2009c).

See also standards 5 and 6 of the HPC (2008) *Standards of conduct, performance and ethics.*

## Delegation

5.2   If you delegate interventions or other procedures you should be satisfied that the person to whom you are delegating is competent to carry them out. In these circumstances, you, as the delegating occupational therapist, retain responsibility for the occupational therapy care provided to the service user (HPC 2008, standard 8).

5.2.1    You should provide appropriate supervision for the individual to whom you have delegated the responsibility.

## Collaborative working

5.3   You should respect the responsibilities, practices and roles of other people with whom you work.

5.3.1   You should be able to articulate the purpose of occupational therapy and the reason for any intervention being undertaken, so promoting the understanding of the profession.

5.3.2   You should recognise the need for multiprofessional and multi-agency collaboration to ensure that well co-ordinated services are delivered in the most effective way.

5.3.3   You have a duty to refer the care of a service user to another appropriate colleague if it becomes clear that the task is beyond your scope of practice. You should consult with other service providers when additional knowledge, expertise and/or support are required (HPC 2008, standard 6).

5.3.4   If you and another practitioner are involved in the treatment of the same service user, you should work co-operatively, liaising with each other and agreeing areas of responsibility. This should be communicated to the service user and all relevant parties.

## Continuing professional development

5.4   You are personally responsible for actively maintaining and continuing your professional development and competence, and for participating in learning opportunities over and above those which are legally required for your work. You must maintain your continuing professional development (CPD) to meet the standards of proficiency for registration with the Health Professions Council.

5.4.1 You are responsible for maintaining a record of your CPD.

5.4.2 You should aim for your CPD to improve the quality of your work and to be of benefit to your service users.

5.4.3 Employing organisations and service managers are encouraged to recognise the value of continuing professional development to individual practitioners, the service and service users.

5.4.4 You should maintain an awareness of current policy, guidelines, research and best available evidence, and should incorporate this into your work where appropriate.

5.4.5 You should be supported in your practice and development through regular professional supervision within an agreed structure or model. Sole practitioners should seek out professional support and advice for themselves.

5.4.6 If you have expert or high-level knowledge, skills and experience, you have a responsibility to share these with your colleagues through supervision, mentoring, preceptorship and teaching opportunities.

More information is available from the *Joint position statement on continuing professional development for health and social care practitioners* (Royal College of Nursing et al 2007) and *Your guide to our standards for continuing professional development* (HPC 2009c).

## Occupational therapy practice education

5.5 You have a professional responsibility to provide regular practice education opportunities for occupational therapy students where possible, and to promote a learning culture within the workplace.

   5.5.1 You should recognise the need for individual education and training to fulfil the role of the practice placement educator. You should, where possible, undertake and maintain accreditation through programmes of study provided by higher education institutions that are recognised by the College of Occupational Therapists.

   5.5.2 If you undertake the role of Practice Placement Educator, you should provide a learning experience for students that complies with the *College of Occupational Therapists pre-registration education standards* (COT 2009e) and the College's current professional standards, and is compatible with the stage of the student's education or training.

   5.5.3 If you accept a student for practice education, you should have a clear understanding of the role and responsibilities of the student, the educational institution and the practice educator.

More information is available from the *College of occupational therapists' curriculum guidance for pre-registration education* (COT 2009d) and the *College of Occupational Therapists pre-registration education standards* (COT 2009e).

# Section Six: Developing and using the profession's evidence base

6.1  As research consumers, you must be aware of the value and importance of research as the basis of the profession's evidence base.

    6.1.1  You should be able to access, understand and critically evaluate research and its outcomes, incorporating it into your practice where appropriate.

    6.1.2  You should audit the services that you provide against appropriate available standards.

    6.1.3  When undertaking any form of research activity, you must understand the principles of ethical research, address the ethical implications and adhere to national and local research governance and ethics requirements.

    6.1.4  When undertaking any form of research activity, you must protect the interests of service users, fellow researchers and others.

    6.1.5  When undertaking any form of research activity, you must protect the confidentiality of participants throughout and after the research process.

6.1.6  When undertaking any form of research activity, you should abide by local, professional and national ethical guidelines and approval processes.

6.1.7  You should disseminate the findings of your research activity through appropriate publication methods in order to benefit the profession and service users, and to contribute to the body of evidence that supports occupational therapy service delivery.

# Appendix 1: Mental capacity

The following is a summary of some of the key, relevant provisions of the *Mental Capacity Act 2005* (Great Britain. Parliament), with references to the *Mental Capacity Act 2005 code of practice* (Department for Constitutional Affairs (DCA) 2007) where appropriate. It is intended to guide you to the relevant parts of the documents, and is not a full statement of the applicable law.

## Mental Capacity Act 2005

Section 1 of the *Mental Capacity Act* (Great Britain. Parliament, Chapter 9) sets out the following principles to be observed when dealing with service users who may lack capacity:

- A person must be assumed to have capacity unless it is established that he (or she) lacks capacity.

- A person is not to be treated as unable to make a decision unless all practicable steps to help him to do so have been taken without success.

- A person is not to be treated as unable to make a decision merely because he makes an unwise decision.

- An act done, or decision made, under this Act for or on behalf of a person who lacks capacity must be done, or made, in his best interests.

■ Before the act is done, or the decision is made, consideration must be given as to whether the desired outcome can be as effectively achieved in a way that is less restrictive of the person's rights and freedom of action.

Section 2 of the Act defines the circumstances in which a person may be said to lack capacity. A person lacks capacity in relation to a situation if, at the particular time, he is unable to make a decision for himself in relation to the situation because of an impairment of, or a disturbance in the functioning of, the mind or brain. Section 2 identifies some factors to be considered when assessing capacity:

■ It does not matter whether the impairment or disturbance is permanent or temporary.

■ A lack of capacity cannot be established merely by reference to:

(a) a person's age or appearance; or

(b) a condition of his, or an aspect of his behaviour, which might lead others to make unjustified assumptions about his capacity.

Section 3 sets out the test for determining whether an individual is unable to make decisions for himself. The *Mental Capacity Act 2005 code of practice* (DCA 2007) states that the assessment of capacity should be undertaken by the person who is directly concerned with the individual at the time the decision needs to be made. That person must assess a service user's capacity to make decisions about his treatment, and may only proceed in the absence of informed consent if they 'reasonably believe' that the individual lacks capacity.

1 For the purposes of Section 2, a person is unable to make a decision for himself if he is unable:

   (a) to understand the information relevant to the decision;

   (b) to retain that information;

   (c) to use or weigh that information as part of the process of making the decision; or

   (d) to communicate his decision (whether by talking, using sign language or any other means).

2 A person is not to be regarded as unable to understand the information relevant to a decision if he is able to understand an explanation of it given to him in a way that is appropriate to his circumstances (using simple language, visual aids or any other means).

3 The fact that a person is able to retain the information relevant to a decision for a short period only does not prevent him from being regarded as able to make the decision.

4 The information relevant to a decision includes information about the reasonably foreseeable consequences of:

   (a) deciding one way or another; or

   (b) failing to make the decision.

If an individual is assessed as lacking capacity, it will be necessary to determine what treatment is in his best interests. There is extensive guidance on this point, but the central points are set out in Section 4 of Chapter 9 of the Act.

Section 5 offers some protection from liability to those involved in the care or treatment of those lacking in capacity. Please refer to the act for further information.

The Social Care Institute for Excellence (SCIE) has developed a web-based *Mental Capacity Act* (Great Britain. Parliament 2005) resource which can be found at:

*http://www.scie.org.uk/publications/mca/index. asp*                    Accessed on 08.03.10.

The Office of the Public Guardian has developed a number of guidance booklets which can be found at:

*http://www.publicguardian.gov.uk/mca/mca.htm*
                    Accessed on 08.03.10.

The *Mental Capacity Act 2005 code of practice* (DCA 2007) is also available from this website.

Practitioners in devolved countries should be aware of their country equivalent legislation and its implications for their practice.

# Appendix 2:
# Informed consent

Anyone over 16 has capacity to consent to treatment and anyone over 18 years has capacity to refuse it. It is to be presumed that a service user has capacity to give informed consent to treatment unless he meets the criteria as set out in Section 2 of the *Mental Capacity Act 2005* (Great Britain. Parliament 2005) (see Appendix 1).

Informed consent is an ongoing agreement by a person to receive treatment, undergo procedures or participate in research, after risks, benefits and alternatives have been adequately explained to them. Informed consent is a continuing requirement. Therefore occupational therapy personnel must ensure that service users continue to understand the information that they have been provided with, and any changes to that information, thereby continuing to consent to the intervention or research in which they are partipating.

If a person cannot communicate their consent, due to disability or injury, it may be possible to infer implied consent if:

■ the service user can reasonably be expected to understand the nature or character of the treatment or procedure; and

- the benefits to the service user outweigh the risks; and

- the service user is given a clear and practical procedure for withholding consent but does not do so.

A service user can only give informed consent if he has the mental capacity to do so. A mentally incapacitated service user cannot validly consent to or refuse treatment, nor can his relatives/carers consent on his behalf. Where a service user lacks the capacity to decide, then under Section 5 of the Act, any treatment is justified if the provider reasonably believes that by giving it, the provider is acting in the best interests of the service user. A number of safeguards apply:

- The practitioner must try to encourage the service user to participate in the decision (Section 4.4).

- The practitioner must consider the service user's past wishes, beliefs and values (prior to the loss of capacity), if these can be ascertained (Section 4.5).

- The practitioner must consider the views of those caring for the service user and anyone else interested in his welfare (Section 4.6).

- The treatment proposed by the practitioner must be proportionate (Section 6.4).

The *Mental Capacity Act 2005* also enables the court to make a decision on behalf of the service user, or appoint a deputy to do so in place of the court (Great Britain. Parliament, Section 16.1(a) and Section 17.1(d)).

# Informed refusal

Informed refusal is a decision not to accept or undergo intervention or participate in research after the risks, benefits and alternatives have been adequately explained.

It is the overriding right of any individual to decide for himself whether or not to accept intervention. Unless a practitioner can rely on the terms of the *Mental Health Act 1983* and the *Mental Capacity Act 2005* (Great Britain. Parliament), they will have committed a trespass to the person if they enforce such intervention, and will be liable to be sued for damages.

The Department of Health has produced numerous guides on consent. These are available at:

> *http://www.dh.gov.uk/en/Publichealth/*
> *Scientificdevelopmentgeneticsandbioethics/*
> *Consent/Consentgeneralinformation/DH_119*
> Accessed on 08.03.10.

Advice relevant to Scotland is available from *A good practice guide on consent for health professionals in the NHSScotland* (Scottish Executive Health Department 2006).

Practitioners in devolved countries should be aware of their country equivalent legislation and its implications for their practice.

# Appendix 3: Information governance

## The Data Protection Act 1998

The *Data Protection Act 1998* (Great Britain. Parliament 1998a) gives individuals the right to know what information is held about them. It provides a framework to ensure that personal information is handled properly.

The Act works in two ways. Firstly, it states that anyone who processes personal information must comply with eight principles, which make sure that personal information is:

- fairly and lawfully processed;
- processed for limited purposes;
- adequate, relevant and not excessive;
- accurate and up to date;
- not kept for longer than is necessary;
- processed in line with peoples' rights;
- secure; and
- not transferred to other jurisdictions without adequate protection.

The second area covered by the Act provides individuals with important rights, including the right to find out what personal information is held about them on computer and most paper records.

The *Data Protection Act 1998* (Great Britain. Parliament 1998a) doesn't guarantee personal privacy at all costs, but aims to strike a balance between the rights of individuals and the sometimes competing interests of those with legitimate reasons for using personal information. It applies to paper records as well as computer records.

## Compliance

The following questions should be considered when dealing with information subject to the *Data Protection Act 1998* (Great Britain. Parliament 1998a). Being able to answer 'yes' to each one does not guarantee compliance and further guidance may be needed, however, answering yes to these questions indicates that compliance with the Act is more likely than not:

- Do I really need this information about an individual? Do I know what I'm going to use it for?

- Do the people whose information I hold know that I've got it, and are they likely to understand what it will be used for?

- If I'm asked to pass on personal information, would the people about whom I hold information expect me to do this?

- Am I satisfied the information is being held securely, whether it's on paper or on computer? And what about my website? Is it secure?

- Is access to personal information limited to those with a strict need to know?

■ Am I sure the personal information is accurate and up to date?

■ Do I delete or destroy personal information as soon as I have no more need for it?

■ Have I trained my staff (or have I been trained) in the duties and responsibilities under the *Data Protection Act 1998* (Great Britain. Parliament 1998a)?

■ Do I need to notify the Information Commissioner and if so is my notification up to date?

Breach of the *Data Protection Act 1998* (Great Britain. Parliament 1998a), or the misuse of information which is subject to the Act, can lead to prosecution and, if convicted of an offence, a fine against a practitioner personally, or his or her employer.

## The Human Rights Act 1998

Article 8 of The European Convention on Human Rights, as incorporated into UK law by the *Human Rights Act 1998* (Council of Europe 1953, Great Britain. Parliament 1998b), provides for the right to respect for private life. Therefore unauthorised disclosure or misuse of personal data will be a breach of an individual's human rights under the Act.

The duty to maintain confidential information ceases in the following circumstances:

■ if the service user gives permission for the information to be disclosed;

■ if the information becomes public by some other means – perhaps the service user publicises it himself; and/or

- if the disclosure of information is 'protected'. This situation would arise if the information disclosed was released as part of a public interest disclosure.

Practitioners in devolved countries should be aware of their country equivalent legislation and its implications for their practice.

# References

*R (Burke) v. General Medical Council (Official Solicitor and others intervening)* [2005] EWCA Civ 1003, [2006] QB 273. Available at: *http://www.familylawweek. co.uk/site.aspx?i=ed409* (paragraph 50)
Accessed on 26.01.10.

Caparo Industries Plc v Dickman [1990] 2 AC 605 (HL).

Christiansen CH, Townsend EA (2004) *Introduction to occupation: the art and science of living.* Upper Saddle River, NJ: Prentice Hall.

College of Occupational Therapists (2002) *From interface to integration: a strategy for modernising occupational therapy services in local health and social care communities. A consultation.* London: COT.

College of Occupational Therapists (2004) *Definition of occupational therapy from member countries, draft 8.* London: COT. Available at: *http://www.wfot. org/office_files/DEFINITIONS%20-%20DRAFT8%20 2007%282%29.pdf*          Accessed on 02.12.09.

College of Occupational Therapists (2006) *Risk management.* London: COT.

College of Occupational Therapists (2007) *Professional standards for occupational therapy practice.* 2nd ed. London: COT.

College of Occupational Therapists (2009a) *Clear sexual boundaries between healthcare professionals and patients: responsibilities of healthcare professionals.* (COT/BAOT Briefings No. 118). London: COT.

College of Occupational Therapists (2009b) *Definitions and core skills for occupational therapy.* (COT/BAOT Briefings No. 23). London: COT.

College of Occupational Therapists (2009c) *Extended scope practice.* (COT/BAOT Briefings No. 14). London: COT.

College of Occupational Therapists (2009d) *The College of Occupational Therapists' curriculum guidance for pre-registration education.* London: COT.

College of Occupational Therapists (2009e) *College of Occupational Therapists pre-registration education standards.* 3rd ed. London: COT.

College of Occupational Therapists (2010) *Record keeping.* 2nd ed. London: COT.

College of Occupational Therapists; Directors of Adult Social Services; Association of Directors of Social Work; Association of Directors for Social Services Cymru (2008) *The value of occupational therapy and its contribution to adult social service users and their carers.* London: COT. Available at: *http://www.cot.org.uk/MainWebSite/Resources/Document/The%20 value%20of%20OT%20and%20its%20contribution.pdf* Accessed on 23.11.09.

Council of Europe (1953) *Convention for the protection of human rights and fundamental freedoms (European convention on human rights) as amended by Protocol No. 11.* Rome: Council of Europe. Available at: *http://conventions.coe.int/treaty/en/Treaties/Html/005.htm* Accessed on 09.03.10.

Creek J (2003) *Occupational therapy defined as a complex intervention.* London: College of Occupational Therapists.

Crepeau EB, Cohn ES, Schell BAB eds (2003) *Willard & Spackman's occupational therapy.* 10th ed. Philadelphia: Lippincott Williams & Wilkins.

Department for Constitutional Affairs (2007) *Mental Capacity Act 2005 code of practice.* London: Stationery Office.

Department of Health (1977) *Relationships between medical and remedial professions.* (HC (77) 33). London: DH.

Department of Health (2009) *Reference guide to consent for examination or treatment.* 2nd ed. London: DH.

Department of Health [ca. 2010a] *Clinical governance.* London: DH. Available at: *www.dh.gov.uk/en/ Publichealth/Patientsafety/Clinicalgovernance/index. htm*                    Accessed on 25.01.10.

Department of Health [ca. 2010b] *Consent key documents.* London: DH. Available at: *http://www. dh.gov.uk/en/Publichealth/ Scientificdevelopmentgeneticsandbioethics/Consent/ Consentgeneralinformation/DH_119*
                                Accessed on 08.03.10.

European Network of Occupational Therapy in Higher Education Terminology Project Group (2004) *Occupational therapy terminology database.* Amsterdam: ENOTHE. Available at: *http://pedit.hio. no/~brian/enothe/terminology/*   Accessed on 25.11.09.

Great Britain. Parliament (1889, 1906, 1916) *Prevention of Corruption Acts 1889 to 1916.* London: HMSO.

Great Britain. Parliament (1974) *Health and Safety at Work Act 1974.* London: HMSO.

Great Britain. Parliament (1983) *Mental Health Act 1983.* London: HMSO.

Great Britain. Parliament (1990) *Access to Health Records Act 1990.* London: HMSO.

Great Britain. Parliament (1995) *Carers (Recognition & Services) Act 1995*. London: HMSO.

Great Britain. Parliament (1998a) *Data Protection Act 1998*. London: Stationery Office.

Great Britain. Parliament (1998b) *Human Rights Act 1998*. London: Stationery Office.

Great Britain. Parliament (1998c) *Public Interest Disclosure Act (PIDA) 1998*. London: Stationery Office.

Great Britain. Parliament (1999) *Health Act 1999*. London: Stationery Office.

Great Britain. Parliament (2000) *Freedom of Information Act 2000*. London: Stationery Office.

Great Britain. Parliament (2005) *Mental Capacity Act 2005*. London. Stationery Office.

Great Britain. Parliament (2006) *Safeguarding Vulnerable Groups Act 2006*. London: Stationery Office.

Hagedorn R (2001) *Foundations for practice in occupational therapy*. 3rd ed. Edinburgh: Churchill Livingstone.

Harvey L (2009) Analytic quality glossary. [s.l]: Quality Research International. Available at: *www.qualityresearchinternational.com/glossary/competence*.htm          Accessed on 25.01.10.

Health Professions Council (2007) *Standards of proficiency: occupational therapists*. London: HPC.

Health Professions Council (2008) *Standards of conduct, performance and ethics*. London: HPC.

Health Professions Council (2009a) *Continuing professional development and your registration*. 2nd ed. London: HPC.

Health Professions Council (2009b) *Guidance on health and character: a guide for applicants and registrants on how we consider information they declare*. London: HPC.

Health Professions Council (2009c) *Your guide to our standards for continuing professional development*. London: HPC.

Health Professions Council (2010) *Guidance on conduct and ethics for students*. London: HPC.

Jameton A, McGuire C (2002) Toward sustainable health-care services: principles, challenges, and a process. *International Journal of Sustainability in Higher Education. 3(2),* 113–127.

Office of the Public Guardian [ca.2010] *[Mental Capacity Act] Forms and Booklets*. Birmingham: OPG. Available at: *http://www.scie.org.uk/publications/mca/index.asp*          Accessed on 08.03.10.

Phillips C, Thompson G (2009) *What is cost effectiveness?* 2nd ed. London: Hayward Medical Communications.

Royal College of Nursing, College of Occupational Therapists, Institute of Biomedical Science (2007) *A joint statement on continuing professional development for health and social care practitioners*. London: RCN.

Scotland: Scottish Executive Health Department (2006) *A good practice guide on consent for health professionals in the NHSScotland*. Edinburgh: Stationery Office.

Social Care Institute for Excellence [ca.2010] *Mental Capacity Act (MCA) resource*. London: SCIE. Available at: *http://www.publicguardian.gov.uk/mca/mca.htm*          Accessed on 08.03.10.

# Bibliography

*Bolitho v City and Hackney Health Authority* [1998] AC 232 (HL).

British Association of Social Workers (2002) *The code of ethics for social workers.* Birmingham: BASW.

British Dietetic Association (2008) *Code of professional conduct.* Birmingham: BDA.

Chartered Society of Physiotherapy (2002) *Rules of professional conduct.* London: CSP.

College of Occupational Therapists (2003) *Research ethics guidelines.* London: COT.

College of Occupational Therapists of Ontario (2009) *Standards for professional boundaries.* Toronto, ON: COTO.

Department of Health (2009) *The NHS constitution: the NHS belongs to us all.* London: DH.

*Donoghue v Stevenson* [1932] AC 562 (HL).

Great Britain. Parliament (1993*) The Access to Health Records (Northern Ireland) Order 1993.* (SI 1250) (NI 4). London: HMSO.

Great Britain. Parliament (2004) *Children Act 2004.* London: Stationery Office.

Professional Foundation of Occupational Therapy in Denmark (2008) *A collection of documents concerning mission, visions, values, professional ethics, cooperation.* Copenhagen, Denmark: Danish Association of Occupational Therapists. Available at: *http://viewer.zmags.com/publication/2639d8ad#/2639 d8ad/1*                                    Accessed on 06.10.09.

Scotland. Scottish Executive (2000) *Adults with Incapacity (Scotland) Act 2000.* Edinburgh: Stationery Office.

Scotland. Scottish Executive (2002) *Freedom of Information (Scotland) Act 2002.* Edinburgh: Stationery Office.

Society and College of Radiographers (2008) *Code of conduct and ethics.* London: SCoR.

Volunteer Development Agency (2009 ) *DIY committee guide common law duty of care help! sheet.* London: Volunteer Development Agency. Available at: *http://www.diycommitteeguide.org/ article/common-law-duty-care-help-sheet*
                                    Accessed on 09.02.10.

World Federation of Occupational Therapists (2005) *Code of ethics.* Forrestfield, AU: WFOT.